Feel Good Now!

When it Comes to Better Health,
There Really is a 'Quick Fix'!

By

Dr. Samuel A Mielcarski, DPT

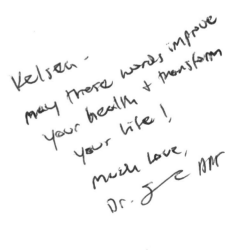

Kelsea -
may these words improve
your health + transform
your life !

much Love,
Dr. J~ DM

DrSamPT Publishing
ISBN-13: 978-1494718169
ISBN-10: 1494718162

DrSamPT.com

Disclaimer

This book is meant for educational purposes only. Under no circumstances should the information contained within this book supersede the instructions given to you by your personal physician or licensed healthcare provider regarding specific conditions for which you are receiving treatment, or have been treated for in the past. You are responsible for your own health and well-being. Neither the author, nor any other co-sponsoring organization and its employees, shall assume or have any responsibility or liability for expenses, medical treatment, or any other forms of compensation for any injury, illness, suffering or discomforts that are experienced as a result of following the information contained within this book.

Okay, now that the legal thing is out of the way, let's get started!

Dedication

This book is dedicated to my parents, Chuck and Linda Mielcarski. I feel so blessed to have grown up in a household where 'principles of health' were emphasized. Thank you so much for these early teachings as they've always stuck with me. It's a privilege and honor to have received the gift of good health; as well as to serve others (including you both) with the guidance in this book. To all of my patients and clients, this work is dedicated to you as well—without you, this book probably would have never been written!

Table of Contents

Preface

You've picked up this book and you're now wondering: 'Is this book right for me?'. Here, let me make the answer to this question really easy for you.

This book IS NOT right for you if:

- You're looking for just another 'magic bullet', 'gimmick', or more 'snake oil' that promises everything in regards to better health, but delivers nothing.
- You believe that you don't actually have to put in any time, spend any money, or do much of anything at all, to improve your health.
- You believe your health is somebody else's responsibility.
- You have no interest at all in improving your health and are not actually going to apply anything that you learn in this book.
- You love being lied to about how to improve your health the right way.
- You plan to use this book as an excuse to avoid improving your health.
- You would rather whine, complain, or blame, instead of taking control of your health.
- You're looking for the answer to be more complicated than it really is when it comes to having better health.
- You want to be told that this book will solve all your health problems.
- You think that you already know all of what is written on the pages of this book and are not open to new learning.

This book IS right for you if:

- You want to end pain and suffering and step into a new and improved vital body.

- You are looking for a doctor brave enough to tell you the truth about how to achieve better health so you can like the person you see in the mirror each day.

- You want to lose weight, have more energy, look younger, and feel better overall.

- You want to stop living on caffeine and other drugs or prescriptions to feel better and just 'get by' in life.

- You want a true 'quick fix' in your health that works both short-term and long-term.

- You want to stop being confused and overwhelmed with complex science and health terminology and would like to learn a simple approach to health that is safe, affordable and easy-to-follow.

- You're tired of being constantly lied to about what it really takes to be healthy.

- You are ready to take responsibility for improving your health, as opposed to just taking magic pills, potions, lotions, and concoctions that don't work.

- You are open to new learning about achieving better health and are willing to be coachable.

- You have made good health a top priority in your life.

So, if this book IS right for you, then buy this book. (If not, then buy it for somebody else.) If you've already bought this book, then congratulations! Let's get started.

Introduction

Are You Ready To *'Feel Good Now'*?

I know you want to improve your health, or at least, you've been thinking about it. How do I know this? I'm psychic. In fact, you can call my psychic healing hotline at: 1-800-DrSam-Psychic-Healer. Seriously, don't call that number. Why? First, I won't answer. Second, it could actually be somebody's number who may not want to hear from you. Bottom line: If you didn't want to improve your health, you wouldn't be reading this book right now.

So, what are you waiting for? I'll bet it's one of the following reasons:

- First reason: You're waiting for permission.
- Second reason: You need some guidance on how to make positive health changes in your life (you need a plan).

If it's the first reason, this shouldn't take long. You have permission to change! There, you are now ready to move forward in your life. Seriously, stop reading this book right now and just go do what you know you should be doing to get the health results you desire. However, if it's the second reason (as it is for many people), this book will provide you with a system of health (Chain-of-Health System™) that you can follow to get positive results. It will teach you how to quickly improve your health, so that you can have a better life. You want the 'quick fix', right? After all, that is why you bought this book. Well, I'm going to teach it to you—I promise!

This book was designed to help you conquer various health challenges such as: pain, low energy levels, depression, poor self-esteem, being overweight, anxiety, high cholesterol, high blood pressure, cancer, diabetes, fibromyalgia, tendinitis, poor posture, and the list goes on. The principles utilized throughout this book are safe, affordable, and easy-to-follow. The information in this book has helped thousands of people of all ages transform their health. Honestly, this book might not just change your life, but even save it!

The results that you get will come down to these two factors:

1. Your willingness to learn. (Trust me. What you'll learn in this book is easy.)
2. Your willingness to change. (Changing your way of thinking and doing.)

Why do many people resist change? It's often because old habits crave attention. The good news is this: *All habits are hard to break, not just the bad ones.* Go back and read that again please. Okay, one more time. So, all you have to do is establish good habits by making small improvements each day and each week and you are bound to succeed!

Your goals are not the end result you desire, but rather what's in front of you. Let me further explain. Your habits (short-term goals) will be the goals you really need to focus on to be successful. This is important. The mistake that many people make when trying to achieve their goals is that too much focus is placed on the goal itself (the long-term goal or end result desired), instead of focusing on the short-term goals—the habits (actions) needed to get there. The problem with this method is that without proper habits, the end result will never be achieved.

For example, if you have a long-term health goal of 'losing 20 pounds', but you don't establish the proper habits necessary to lose the weight, you're not going to be successful. Many people with weight-loss goals are too focused on stepping on the scale every day to see if they are 'there yet', instead of making the necessary diet and lifestyle changes to actually get there. The bottom line: The weight won't come off unless you do what's needed to get it off—no matter how many times a day you step on the scale!

Some people refer to habits or goals as 'standards of living' instead. It doesn't matter what you call them, the key is that you're focused on taking action by changing them (your habits and/or standards of living).

This is how you will succeed. This can be applied to any goal in life. I will give you some guidance throughout this book about what actions you need to take, or what new standards you need to live by, to achieve your health goals.

Small steady improvements will lead to large changes in your health over time. Consider this: as little as a 2% improvement per week can lead to a 100% improvement by the end of one year. Let's do some simple math: 2% improvement x 52 weeks in a year = 104% improvement! (My math is off a bit, huh? Not really. I'm just giving you 2 weeks off for good behavior.) So, do you think you can manage a 2% improvement in your health each week? Is that really too much to ask of yourself? Of course not. I know you can do this!

A Simple Approach To Health

There are two main ways to approach your health. You can either focus on promoting wellness, or you can focus on disease management. The first way is proactive, preventive, affordable and easy to understand. The second way is reactive, palliative, expensive and difficult to understand. After comparing the two approaches to health, it makes sense to choose the first way, which is the focus of this book.

The Cost Of Health vs. The Cost Of Sickness

Every way I've ever analyzed it (financially, physically, emotionally, spiritually, environmentally, etc.), the cost of health is always less than the cost of sickness. For example, the cost of this book is far less than you'd pay for an hour with a rehabilitation specialist, doctor, or 'healer' almost anywhere in the United States. In fact, it's probably much less expensive than what you may already be paying weekly for medications, therapies, or various healing methods (that often don't even work). You only paid for this book one time (or you may have even received it for free), but for the rest of your life, you'll have a resource that will be worth hundreds or even thousands of times its cost—in your health! Being sick or injured isn't fun, and it's not affordable either. Do you know what a new liver would cost you? Tens of thousands of dollars. Now, that's expensive! However, instead of cutting out and replacing bad body parts, this book will teach you how to cut out and replace bad habits instead.

Mother Nature Is NOT Prejudiced!

After restoring my own health, as well as helping thousands of people overcome various health challenges, I came to a significant conclusion: 'Mother Nature is NOT prejudiced!' What exactly does this mean? This means that she doesn't care what color you are, how old you are, your gender, how much you weigh, where you live, your eye color, etc. The rules are the rules! So, the good news is that there's hope for you! You just have to be willing to follow some simple rules. Since you might not like the concept of rules, let's just call them *guidelines* instead. If you struggle with change, don't worry; this book can help you. People often fear change. They fear it because they don't want to fail. The whole thing is really silly because change is going to happen whether you like it or not. You only fail when you fail to act and not do what's in your best interest. So, guess what? If you follow the guidance in this book, you really can't fail!

Why People Struggle To Fix Their Health (The 'Holy Grail Syndrome')

The biggest reason people don't take charge of their health is that they don't know where to begin. Always remember: *Begin with the basics*. If people don't understand the basics, then they usually won't do anything at all (at least not for the long-term). Consequently, many people end up suffering from what I like to call: 'The Holy Grail Syndrome'. This occurs when a person keeps looking for, and chasing after, what is believed to be the 'Holy Grail of Health'—that one thing that will fix all of their health problems! For some, it's that one magic food. For some, it's that one magic pill or supplement. For others, it's a special concoction or spiritual practice from antiquity. Or, it may even be about finding that almighty guru that will give them the secrets of the universe. The irony is that they will spend a ton of time, money, and energy in search of the

'Holy Grail', while continually ignoring the simple basics needed to build better health that are right in front of them. Then, when this Holy-Grail-approach fails, they may finally consider trying to apply some of these health basics correctly. This approach seems backwards, doesn't it? Don't worry though, this book won't be about another Holy-Grail-approach, but rather about you learning the basics of health needed to feel good quickly.

Why 'Feel Good Now'?

When feeling good, you're going to perform at your best in life. You'll be a better father, mother, brother, sister, athlete, student, musician, artist, etc. When feeling good, you will help others in need. When feeling good, you will live with more passion and purpose. When feeling good, you're likely to act with more compassion, be more patient, have more tolerance, give more and take less, smile more, laugh more and enjoy your life...more! So, when is the best time to feel good? *Now!* Not tomorrow, next week, next year or somewhere down the road, but right now! Why would you want to wait? You have to live in the now. So, now is the best time to feel good! When you get into the habit of feeling good now, that's when your health will be transformed quickly.

Keep reading...

Chapter 1

Four Simple Health Lessons To Help You Feel Better Fast!

My parents have been two of the best coaches I've ever had in my life. The topic of health was just one of the many things they helped coach me on. I was blessed to grow up in a household where health principles were taught and emphasized. However, I have to admit, I didn't always listen. Suffice it to say, some of these lessons were painful. Honestly, it wasn't until I was a young adult faced with serious health challenges that my parents' early teachings really served me well—they saved my life! So, let us begin with four simple lessons to help you better understand how to improve your health quickly.

Lesson 1: The 'Art Of Health' vs. The 'Science Of Health'

There is an important difference between the 'art of health' and the 'science of health'. If you take nothing from this book except this one simple five-word-phrase, then you will probably be way ahead of where you were before you picked up this book. This phrase will promote and reinforce positive health changes in your life. I like to call it the 'Golden Health Mantra'. Here it is: *Health comes from healthy living*. Let me repeat that: *Health comes from healthy living*.

This sounds so simple, right? When feeling well, this phrase seems to make perfect sense. However, when not feeling well, you may develop amnesia quickly and forget how to take care of yourself. Here, let me remind you: *Except in extreme cases where some kind of necessary emergency medical care may be needed, the factors that make one well are the same as the factors that keep one well*. The 'art of health' is a need-to-know concept. Whenever in doubt, always follow the 'art of heath'. This can help you avoid information overload, or over-complicating health matters; as well as help you avoid bogus health schemes, scams, or the next greatest over-hyped cure known to mankind. Again, the 'art of health' is really simple: *Health comes from healthy living*.

Conversely, the 'science of health' is very complicated. It can lead people down a never-ending path or quest for answers; and ironically enough, it often leads to less than optimal results most of the time. The 'science of health' tries to micro-manage everything. Although it's fun to learn about the human body, these things are a nice-to-know concept, but that's what books are for. You don't need an eight-year degree from some prestigious university or understand big words, such as, hypothalamic-pituitary-adrenal axis, to be healthy. Yeah, it may sound cool, but we are talking health here, not Fonzi from Happy Days. (Correct-a-mundo!)

Since we live in a modern day world of so-called 'evidence-based health practice', I often hear people say, "Show me the science!", when it comes to something that might benefit their health. When I hear this, a great Eastern proverb comes to mind: *"When a man's science exceedth his sense, he perishes by ignorance"*. Science can often be manipulated and flawed. Besides, all the true science usually ever does is validate the art anyway. For example, 'Study X' shows that some simple requisite of good health (such as one of the various factors within the Chain-of-Health System™) is actually good for you. Don't get trapped in the complex science; just follow the simple art instead!

Key takeaway: Keep health matters simple and you'll succeed. Just stick to the basics. Remember: *Health comes from healthy living*. This is the 'art of health'.

Lesson 2: Knowledge vs. Wisdom

There is an important difference between knowledge and wisdom. Knowledge is knowing, and wisdom is doing. I've met many people in my life that have an incredible amount of health knowledge. They know everything there is to know about health (or, at least they think they do). I can't tell you how many times I've heard people say, "I already know all of this.", when being coached on the topic of health. However, these are often the same people who aren't doing what they proclaim to know. They usually have a huge disconnect between what they think they're doing, and what they're actually doing. For example, to know that eating fruits and veggies as part of a healthy diet is NOT the same as actually eating them!

These well-meaning health seekers often pursue all knowledge, but master none of it. Consequently, they end up with poor health as well. In order to be good at something, you must practice. If you want better health, you must practice better health. Each day, you can practice better health by becoming more aware of your body, making healthier choices, and implementing simple health habits or strategies. After all, you can only experience good health to the degree to which you practice it!

Key takeaway: When it comes to feeling better, if you don't do it, you really don't know it.

Lesson 3: Health Is Earned!

What motivates people to have better health? Two things: *rewards* and *pain*. Let's first discuss rewards. People want to be rewarded for their efforts. They want to see and feel the results. If you follow the Chain-of-Health System™ outlined in this book, you will get the results you desire. However, the best way to follow this system is without regard for the rewards. This is the highest level of devotion and will move you much faster towards your main goal—feeling good now! Let's now discuss pain. Most people don't like pain, especially the kind of pain and suffering associated with not feeling well. Pain is a strong stimulus that can motivate change. When pain becomes great enough in one's life to change (so that the pain is no longer felt), then change will occur. This may be one reason why you're reading this book right now. You've reached your pain threshold, so you're now ready to do what it takes to change your health and end the suffering!

The petals of a flower open as a result of the sun hitting it, not because they are forced open. You can't force better health. Remember, it's a result of healthful living—*health is earned!* Whether it's good health or poor health, either way, health is earned. If you currently have poor health, it didn't happen overnight; only your awareness of it might have.

In other words, it took time to acquire poor health, and it will take some time to correct it. However, there really is a 'quick fix'. Your daily actions will determine what direction your health moves in. If you participate in the causes of good health, you will have good health. Conversely, participating in the causes of poor health will lead to poor health.

Key takeaway: Good or bad, health is earned!

Lesson 4: Knowing Where to Start: Assess Don't Guess!

There is a premise in the world of rehabilitation: *If you're not assessing, then you're just guessing.* Well, unless you're a really lucky person, guessing usually doesn't get the job done well. As a rehabilitation specialist and wellness consultant, I choose to work only with people that will agree to be assessed first. How can the right treatment be rendered if no assessment is ever done? Answer: It can't! Unfortunately, this happens all too often though. If you want to figure out the best way to fix something quickly (and correctly), you first need to figure out what's wrong with it. Your health is no exception!

Before beginning any type of regimen to improve your health, you should perform some type of assessment. This will not only help you find the best way to go about improving your health quickly, it will also help you avoid wasting your precious time, money, and energy trying to figure it all out as you go. Having a plan that is based on some type of assessment is one of the biggest keys to getting a 'quick fix'! You'll learn more about this in the next chapter.

Key takeaway: Knowing where to start will make it much easier to end up where you want to go quickly. Take the time to assess first.

Chapter 2

Your Chain-of-Health System™:
The Real 'Quick Fix!'

Okay, let's get into why you really bought this book. You want results and you want them now! Go ahead, say it! Say it! Say it: "I want the quick fix!" There, you said it. Feel better yet? As the subtitle of this book reads: *When it comes to better health, there really is a 'quick fix!'* So, are you ready for the big secret no one is telling you? Okay, here it is: If you find and fix the weakest link in your health first, then you'll get the 'quick fix'!

There's an old saying: "A chain is only as strong as its weakest link." Well, it's no different with your health. You have a Chain-of-Health System™. If you strengthen the weakest link in your Chain-of-Health System™ first, this will be the fastest way to better health—you'll get the 'quick fix'! There will be a total of eight 'health links' discussed in this book. All good coaches teach and reinforce the basics. Your job is to master the basics by learning about the eight links. My job is to teach them to you. After all, the word 'doctor' means teacher. (Yes, you can call me 'Coach Sammy' if you like.)

Key Points:

1. Your health is only as strong as its weakest link.
2. The fastest way to better health is to find and fix the weakest link first.

The Chain-of-Health System™

The essential eight links in the Chain-of-Health System™ that will be discussed in this book are as follows: Food-Air-Water-Light-Rest-Activity-Hygiene-Love. Each of the next eight chapters of this book will be dedicated to addressing one of these links so that you will better understand each link in greater detail, as well as how to fix a link when and if it's weak. It's important to understand that the Chain-of-Health

System™ works both short-term and long-term. In other words, it can help you feel good now, as well as feel better overall in the future.

A Quick Note About How This Book Came About

When I first wrote this book, it was very long and had a great deal of information in it. I kept reading and revising it until I pared it down to what I thought was a reasonable amount of information that most people would be willing to start with. Although each link in the Chain-of-Health System™ is easy to understand, there is much depth to each of them. The focus of this book isn't to cover this depth, but rather focus on one key takeaway for each link that most people would be willing to follow to feel good now! With that said, if you would like to explore the Chain-of-Health System™ in greater depth, you can check out some of the other products and services that I have available. (For more information, please visit: DrSamPT.com) For now, keep reading.

A Simple Assessment

I carry my own business card in my pocket each day. The Chain-of-Health System™ is written on the back of it. If, or when, I need to feel better, I take out the card, look at the Chain-of-Health System™ and ask myself: "What's missing right now?" One of the links usually jumps out at me (Not literally, but that would be a cool business card if it did, huh?). This link is then addressed at that moment in the day and my health is transformed immediately. Many of my patients and clients have found this simple assessment useful as well. You may have even received a card with the Chain-of-Health System™ on it with the purchase of this book. (Note: You can get a card by visiting FeelGoodNowTheBook.com. Enter bonus code: FGN8)

So, how will you know which link(s) may need immediate attention in your Chain-of-Health System™ to help you feel good now? First, nobody is perfect, so there is always room for improvement somewhere in the chain. So, now that we have your ego in check and have enlightened you about your less than God-like status, let's continue pondering this

14

question of how to determine where your Chain-of-Health System™ needs to be strengthened. Said another way: How will you know where to start?

The answer is: Sometimes you'll just know and sometimes you won't. For example, when you review the links in the Chain-of-Health System™ (Food-Air-Water-Light-Rest-Activity-Hygiene-Love), one of them will stand out to you. It will call to you. If the link could speak, here's what it might say: "Here I am." "Yo, right here!" "Hello darling, I'm the one you've been looking for." "Fix me first, please." "Dude, what's up? Are we going to do this or what?" "Hello, it's about time." "Hey, could you give me some help over here." Okay, I'm sure you get the idea. So, sometimes you'll just already know where to begin. When this happens, it makes the whole process easier.

So, you may be thinking to yourself right now, "Well, that's just great! Some people receive a get-out-of-jail-free-card, huh? What about those of us that just still don't know where to start? What if a link doesn't scream at me or jump off the card and say: 'Here I am!'? What the heck do I do then? Huh? Huh?" Okay, calm down. Don't panic. I got you covered my little health seeker. All you need to do is just rate each of the links on a scale from 1-10 (with 1 being the lowest score and 10 being the highest). The link with the lowest score is the weakest link—and should be addressed immediately if you want the 'quick fix' to help you feel good now! So, how do you actually score each link? If you have addressed a link adequately for the day, it would get a higher score (7-10 for example). If you have addressed a link partially, but not adequately, it would get a middle-range score (4-6 for example). If you haven't addressed a link at all, it would get a low-range score (0-3 for example). With practice, you'll get better at identifying your body's true needs and using this simple rating system. Yes, one day, you may even join the ranks of others in the 'Weakest-Link-Just-Jumps-Off-The-Card-At-Me Club'. (This is a very prestigious club by the way.) Okay, now that you have a simple way to assess yourself, let's keep going.

Your Mindset

What you tell yourself over and over again will eventually come true. So, as opposed to saying or focusing on the fact that you have a 'weak link', your mindset needs to be on the idea of 'all links are strong' instead. This way, your words, thoughts, and actions will be towards strong and vibrant health, as opposed to focusing on having weak health. You should also refer to any 'weak link' as a 'key link' in your Chain-of-Health System™. This particular mindset about the links is very important to your success.

Throughout this book, I'm going to provide you with little sayings and phrases to help you reprogram your mind. Each of the eight links will have some of these key phrase reminders—'Link Builders'—to help you succeed in improving your health. Now, let's get to addressing those essential eight links, shall we?

Chapter 3

Link #1- Food
'Fast Food' Is Good For You!

What if I told you that 'fast food' is good for you? Hard to believe, huh? Believe it; because it's true! You can (and should) eat 'fast food', especially if you want to feel good now! However, notice I said 'fast food', not junk food. There is a significant difference. What many people call 'fast food' is just really junk food. Junk food often comes in a package, bag or box (usually full of salt, grease, fat, sugar, and many preservatives) and may be obtained by placing an order for it by speaking through a clown's mouth or some other crazy looking microphone. It does come fast. Most people eat it fast. They pollute their body fast. Then, they feel really lousy—fast! This type of food is more of a modern-day inconvenience, as opposed to a convenience. It has some superficial appeal, but it lacks the deep nutritional value needed to truly build better health. Bottom line: If you eat junk, then you will feel like junk!

Real 'fast food' is a bit different though. This type of food doesn't have a long list of harmful ingredients attached to it. It does sometimes come in a package, but it's usually just the one that nature has made for it. It comes in multiple colors and is very visually tantalizing to the eye. Its aroma is very fresh and uplifting. Its texture feels pleasurable. It sounds good (it doesn't cry out or fight back). Its flavor is heavenly with universal appeal. It's often easy to find and is very affordable in most places. So, what's this real 'fast food' I'm speaking of? The answer is: *produce!*

Here's another way of looking at it. There are basically two types of food a person can eat when wanting to feel better quickly: *produce* or *reduce*. You may have heard of produce before. It's often called fresh (organic) fruits and vegetables. There are other types of produce as well, such as: nuts, seeds, sprouts, legumes, tubers, herbs, grasses, grains, and wild edibles. Now, let's discuss reduce. That would be the other stuff, especially processed junk foods such as: refined carbohydrates (starches, chips, bread products, high fructose corn syrup, or sugars), genetically modified foods, foods containing pesticides, herbicides or fungicides, artificial sweeteners, hydrogenated fats and oils, protein powders, factory-farmed and processed meats (burgers, hotdogs, chicken and pig parts, etc.), homogenized and pasteurized dairy products, and food dyes, colorings and other additives. Simply put, reduce *is*, and *does*, the opposite of produce. So, the choice is yours: 'Fast food' (produce) or junk food (reduce)?

Feel-Alive Foods

If there's not life in your food, then why have food in your life? Your food needs to be 'alive' in order for you to feel alive. What does this mean? It means that the more your food is processed and treated, the less potential it has to supply you with the vital nutrients and energy your body needs to be healthy and feel good now! It just makes sense that life begets life. (Live food = live cells, and dead food = dead cells.) So, if you want to feel whole, natural and alive, it would only make sense to eat more whole, natural and living foods (fresh produce), especially organic fruits and veggies. Here's some ancient wisdom from an old book that indicates this might be a good idea also: "*Then God said, Behold, I have given you every plant yielding seed that is on the surface of all the earth, and every tree which has fruit yielding seed; it shall be food for you.*" (Genesis 1:29) So, eating 'fast food' (produce) appears to have been a divine plan as well.

"Don't dig your grave with your own knife and fork."
-old English proverb

More On 'Fast Food' To Help You Feel Better

Okay, now that you know the truth that 'fast food' is good for you, let's discuss it in a bit more detail to help you understand how to consume it in a way to help you feel better. The more complex the food you eat, the harder it will be to digest your food. The more energy that gets put into digestion, the less energy you will have for other things, such as feeling good now! We do live in a fast-paced world. We have responsibilities, commitments and goals to achieve. The foods we eat can support this lifestyle, but this is only going to happen correctly if you make the right food choices. Otherwise, you will feel the drain, as many do, after they eat.

The task of digestion requires a good deal of energy, especially when eating the wrong kinds of foods. Have you ever wondered why so many people feel tired and sometimes even fall asleep after eating? (By the way, while common, this isn't normal.) Their energy is being zapped because most of it is going into the task of trying to digest all that has been eaten. As a result, the body shuts down (slows down or falls asleep) to conserve energy to allow digestion to occur. If the body didn't perform this act of self-preservation, then it could be the last meal one ever eats!

Therefore, if you want to improve your energy levels significantly, you must improve your digestion. One easy way to improve your digestion is to just simplify your meals by not eating too many different things at once. For example, consider making a meal out of just a few different kinds of organic fruits and veggies. It's really not hard to do. Just pick one kind up and eat it until you've had enough. Then, move on to the next kind. When you think about it, nothing is really faster than that! Another convenient way to consume produce is to turn it into a smoothie—there are so many delicious options!

Not So 'Fast'!

Sometimes, in order to speed up your results, you have to slow down a bit. In other words, you need to take some time and eat mindfully. Mindful eating includes chewing your food adequately. Whether it's food or drink, anything consumed should be adequately mixed with your saliva to maximize digestion and improve your energy levels. This saying may help you: '*Drink your food and chew your drink. This will prevent it from being a weak link!*' Eating mindfully also encompasses being present and not trying to multi-task while eating. If your body is too busy doing too many other things, it can't be digesting too well. If you want to feel good now, then you have to be in the now!

19

*Bonus: Learn a simple exercise that will help you determine how well you chew. Visit: FeelGoodNowTheBook.com. Enter bonus code: FGN8

Real Hunger

Many people have lost touch with what true hunger and satiation (being full) really feel like. True hunger is usually not painful, and it isn't felt deep in the stomach region and accompanied by some weird gurgling noises. This experience is often a sign of dehydration, or intestinal distress (meaning something doesn't need to go into the body, but rather come out). True hunger is a sure and definite feeling that is often a pleasant, hollow and throaty feeling. In other words, you shouldn't be confused about whether or not you should eat. If you think that you're hungry, then you're probably not! Hunger is a definitive yes or no; not a maybe. If you're truly hungry, you won't have to think about it. You'll be sure. However, you may need to get used to this new hunger awareness, which can take some practice.

Have you ever had this experience? You think that you're hungry because your stomach is talking to you with some noises and a bit of discomfort and your energy levels are running low. So, you figure it must be time to eat, right? However, you wait long enough and the feelings go away and your energy levels go up and you immediately feel better. What happened? What you were experiencing wasn't true hunger. True hunger will persist—and nothing will satisfy this need except eating. So, when unsure, then just follow this simple guideline: *When in doubt, just wait it out, as true needs (such as hunger) will always persist.*

Okay, now that you understand what hunger is, let's discuss how being full is supposed to feel. Being full (satiated) should be a feeling of satisfaction without any discomfort or negative side effects. It shouldn't hurt, feel like you are stuffed and going to explode, or make you want to fall asleep; nor should it create gas, bloating, or other discomforts. These symptoms have become so common after eating that many people believe they are normal. Nature didn't intend to punish us daily for fulfilling a basic survival need (eating). This just doesn't make sense, does it?

The Clock Says It's Time to Eat

Our bodies run on a natural biological clock that dictates when you should eat. This is the clock that is inside of you, not the one that may be strapped to your wrist or hanging on the wall. There is a time of the day when digestive capacity is best. This is when there is natural light available. So, if you need a light to see what you're eating, you probably shouldn't be eating it. This means that eating late at night, especially right before (within a couple of hours of) bedtime is not wise. Doing so will encroach upon the time the body is trying to do other important things at night, such as heal and recover. Part of the secret to feeling good now is doing things that help you feel good later—not eating late is one of them! Keep eating matters simple: Eat by day, rest by night. As a general guideline, eating should usually cease two hours before going to bed.

Food As A Reward

Food is often used as a reward. Is this really a good idea? It depends. It's a good idea if it's being used to reward the right thing—true hunger! If you want food to reward a 'job well done' or some other kind of personal accomplishment, then just make sure you've earned it. Make sure that you're truly hungry. It's okay to celebrate with food. Just consider what you're truly celebrating; the fact that you're hungry, and nothing but that. Using food as a reward for anything else (but true hunger) is not recommended. It will inevitably lead to an unhealthy relationship with food.

Okay, let's summarize:

1. Eat real 'fast food'- fresh (raw & organic) fruits and veggies or other produce.
2. Eat simple meals to improve digestion- avoid eating too many things at one time.

3. Eat mindfully- be present, just eat, and take the time to chew your food.
4. Eat only when truly hungry and stop when full.

The following 'Link Builder' may help you stay on track when your 'Food Link' needs attention. Reading or saying this phrase often can serve as a nice reminder about the importance of proper nutrition to feel good now!

Link Builder: **To feel good now and thrive, eat the 'fast foods' that are alive!**

Chapter 4

Link #2- Air
Getting 'High' On Life Force!

Besides wholesome food, air is another very important nutrient that you will need to feel good now! There are two main concepts that should be considered regarding the 'Air Link': the quality of how you breathe; and the quality of air you breathe. This chapter will primarily address the quality of how you breathe.

Here is a quick assessment for you to perform:

Step 1: Sit facing a mirror, one hand on your chest and one on your stomach.

Step 2: Looking in the mirror, focus your eyes at the top of your shoulder region.

Step 3: Take in a deep breath.

Step 4: Notice what the top of your shoulders do?

Did your chest-hand rise first and your shoulders move up toward your ears? If yes, then this means you're an 'upper chest breather'. This also means that you're probably only using about one-third of your total lung capacity, which isn't very much. Said another way, this also means that you're cutting off your life force energy by approximately seventy percent!

Conversely, when you took that breath in, if your shoulders hardly moved upward at all and the hand on your stomach moved (outward and upward) first, then congratulations, as you're most likely breathing correctly—breathing more fully by using your diaphragm muscle, instead of your neck, chest and shoulder muscles to breathe. This means more life force energy moving through you more often, which means feeling good now, more often.

When I explored the concept of breathing in depth, I remember a teacher telling me: *"How you breathe is how you live."* What does this mean? It means that if your breath is tight and restricted, your life will probably feel like that also. This may result in you feeling anxious all the time; or tired, or tense and tight in your body. It's one thing to understand this concept, but it's another to truly experience it. If you're willing to explore your breathing a bit further, you can experience what I'm talking about.

"Whoever nourishes himself with air becomes radiant like a god and lives a long life." -Confucius

Do this little exercise now:

Step 1: Sit or lie down in a quiet, safe place.
Step 2: Breathe slowly and deeply (breathing in four seconds, and out four seconds.)
Step 3. Start thinking about something that makes you happy or joyful. Notice what happens to your breathing.
Step 4: Start thinking about something that makes you scared or angry and upset. Again, notice what happens to your breathing.

When your thoughts were on happiness and joy, was your breath free and deep? How about being angry or scared? Did your breathing become restricted and shallow? If you're not sure, do the exercise again. If you're sure, it's pretty amazing, huh? Yes, your thoughts help to shape your emotions, which in turn help to dictate how your body functions (your physiology). So, just by changing your thoughts, you can change how you breathe. The good news is that the opposite is true as well. If you breathe full and deep, you can change how you think and how you feel immediately!

One of the simplest ways to feel better using breath is to just let it out. For example, have you ever noticed how good a 'sigh' feels? It's as though all of your problems have been expelled in one nice breath! The 'ahhh' or 'heee' or whatever other noise you make just seems to help all your worries and stress go away. Although it's important to take a 'breath of relief' when needed, it's just as important to 'breathe well' the rest of the time so you don't even get to this point to begin with. Cultivating breath awareness is key. Your body will send you clear signals, so just pay attention. Remember: *"How you breathe is how you live."* So, if you're not feeling the way you want to, consider changing how you're breathing.

As I've said earlier, and probably will again at some point in this book: 'Mother Nature is NOT prejudiced!' Therefore, if you choose not to breathe into your life, you won't have much life at all—it will lack energy, and your life may eventually be significantly shortened (expire) as well. Air is vital for sure. When compared to food and water, air is usually the least valued and yet, the most important. Consider this: You can probably live weeks and months without food, days without water, but only minutes without air!

A Good Return On Your Investment

If I were going to recommend at least one health changing habit for you to follow, it would be to improve your breathing awareness and function! Read that one again. Okay, again. Again, please. Breathing can have so many profound positive effects on so many levels. You will know what I'm talking about once you actually incorporate this new health practice (correct breathing) into your life. If you need some extra motivation, how about a reward on your time and energy invested? Remember: Health is earned! So, you will have to invest some in your health. When looking at any aspect of health, you should always consider what your ROI will be (ROI = Return on Investment). Would you be more likely to invest in your health if you knew the reward was going to be great? Of course you would!

Well, then consider this: You breathe approximately twenty thousand times per day on average. So, would it make sense that any small improvement in your breathing would yield huge returns? Let me help you: 'YES', it would! With improved breathing awareness and practice, your breathing efficiency will improve. This means that you will take fewer breaths per minute to achieve the same or even better health results than before. Healthier people tend to breathe less, but get more—feel good now!

Breathing Better x 20,000x /day = FEELING MUCH BETTER!

Bonus: Learn how a simple piece of string can help you become a better breather. Visit: FeelGoodNowTheBook.com. Enter bonus code: FGN8

General Benefits Of Breathing

Breath cleanses and strengthens the physical, emotional and spiritual aspects of your body. Said another way, breathing properly can help to:

- improve blood and lymph flow (improve circulation).
- cleanse and detoxify the body (remove large amounts of toxins).
- improve mental clarity (think and concentrate better).
- enhance emotional well-being (great anti-depressant).
- improve self-confidence (improve self-image).
- change limiting beliefs and behaviors.
- decrease pain and muscle tension (great analgesic and anti-inflammatory).
- increase connection with higher spiritual realms (God-consciousness).
- improve sleep (rejuvenate and heal the body, mind and soul).
- improve sexual functioning (physically, mentally and spiritually).
- enhance digestion and elimination.
- improve posture and alignment.
- improve overall mobility and strength.
- improve self-awareness.
- reconnect one to the present moment.
- AND MUCH MORE...

'Breathing Check-ups' May Be Needed

When trying to improve your breathing habits, you may need to perform a 'breathing check-up' (or 'check in') with yourself. How often? As much as it takes—although you shouldn't get obsessed with this task. Checking in with yourself several times a day wouldn't be too much. When are you supposed to do this? Just simply fit it into your normal routine. You could tag it along with something else that is routine in your life. For example, you could use some of the red lights (while in traffic) as a 'breath check-up' opportunity. You could 'check in' when listening to someone talk to you (breathe deeply and listen well). 'Checking in' every time you go to the bathroom (which should be several times a day by the way) would be another opportunity. Other times may be while you're in the shower, before bed, or before eating. Your options are many. You could also set yourself up some reminders. A note that says 'breath check' placed at your computer or on the screen saver, on the fridge, in the bathroom, at work, or near your bed. As simple as this is, it really works. It works well; but only if you do it!

How To Breathe

When you're not speaking, engaging in intense exercise or physical activity, or performing some kind of special breathing exercise, breathing through your nose versus your mouth is recommended. Breathing through your nose will help warm and filter the air as you take it into your body. It also allows the air to be mixed with a gas inside the nose that is called nitric oxide, which helps your lungs absorb oxygen better. Nose breathing may also help keep you calm and focused, whereas if you are a mouth dominant breather, you may find that you have a harder time relaxing and staying focused, as well as maintaining good posture.

Sometimes, just having a simple reminder can help you stay on track to improve your health. The following is a simple breathing reminder: 'Breathe low, slow, and through the nose with lips closed.' This reminder could be placed in several locations where you'll see it throughout your day to help cue you to not only breathe, but to breathe correctly.

'Breathing low' means breathing from your diaphragm (lower abdomen), as opposed to your upper chest, neck, and shoulders. 'Breathing slow' means breathing deep and calmly, as opposed to shallow and quickly. 'Breathing through the nose with lips closed' means breathing through your nose, as opposed to breathing through an open mouth.

Air Quality

So far, we've discussed the quality of how you breathe. Now, let's discuss the quality of air that you breathe. One of the simplest ways to ensure good air quality is to avoid polluting the air you're breathing! This should be common sense. However, I have seen many people not only become accustomed to poor air quality, they unfortunately contribute to it as well. When you consider the way people often perform the acts of cooking, cleaning, leisure tasks, and basic hygiene and self-care, it's really amazing how many times a day people actually pollute the very air they're trying to breathe! (I think we are the only species that does this by the way.)

Another great way to improve air quality is to just allow more 'fresh air' into your living space. This may mean opening a window, turning on a fan, going outside, or using an air purifier if needed. By the way, plants make great air purifiers. (They are cheap, energy efficient, quiet, environmentally safe, low maintenance and esthetically pleasing.) Some other simple measures would be to: stop smoking, avoid smoke-filled environments, don't burn paraffin candles, use only natural and environmentally friendly self-care and housecleaning products, as well as natural building materials and home furnishings. Keeping your living and working space clean and orderly will help improve air quality also.

The following 'Link Builder' will help you address your 'Air Link' when it needs attention. Reading or saying this phrase often can serve as a nice reminder about the importance of proper breathing to feel good now!

Link Builder: **Breathe low, slow, and through the nose with lips closed!**

Chapter 5

Link #3- Water
Your 'Drinking Habit' Could Be Draining You!

Life on this planet depends on water; and so does your health! Both the human body and the body of Mother Earth are composed mostly of water; not mostly of energy drinks, diet drinks, tea, coffee, alcohol, soda, milk, or sports drinks. Water is a wise drink of choice if one wishes to be healthy. Not only is water the primary constituent of all body fluids, it's also responsible for holding us together at the cellular level and gives rise to our very shape and form overall. Water also plays a role in producing and storing energy within the body.

Water helps to purify the body. It does this by not only being a strong solvent, but also being a perfect solution as well. This solution acts as a delivery system bringing nutrients to, and waste products away from, cells. Most, if not all, physiologic functions of the body are dependent upon water. It may be considered good medicine too, as water is what helps guide natural healing processes to occur. Therefore, if you want to have more energy, stay healthy, and feel good now, you must avoid chronic dehydration, which is very common in many people.

> *"I believe that water is the only drink for a wise man."*
> -Henry David Thoreau

When it comes to water, both quantity and quality are important. Let's first discuss quantity—or how much? How much water should you consume? The answer is: *enough*. This means that the amount of water you need on a daily basis can change. It will depend on many factors, such as these physiological factors: height, weight, body composition (body fat vs. lean muscle), genetic predisposition, and metabolic rate. Your overall fitness level and hydration status can also determine your water needs. The following environmental factors can affect hydration as well: one's activity level (intensity and duration of work or sport), climate (temperature and acclimation to it), and the amount of clothing or equipment that may be used during activities. Therefore, the right amount of water on any given day just depends on your needs.

Since *enough* may not be something that you can totally comprehend, let me give you a general guideline. On average, one may lose up to three to four liters of water each day via bowel and bladder elimination, sweating and breathing. If this water isn't replaced adequately, dehydration may result and health can suffer. Also, for every hour of exercise or intense physical activity, half to one liter of water may need to be consumed. So, it would make sense to at least replace what is being lost each day. Consuming too much water can result in 'water intoxication' (which happens very rarely) and leads to ill health. Although proper hydration is desired, there is no need to flood your insides out!

Preventing Dehydration

One way to prevent dehydration is to avoid consuming 'water robbers'. A 'water robber' is a term that I made up to describe something that causes your body to need and/or utilize more water. For example, over-cooked food is really food that's dehydrated—as much of the water (as well as other nutrients, such as minerals) that help to ensure proper hydration has been removed. This type of food can act like a sponge inside the body drawing on the body's water supply. This is one more reason to include plenty of fresh, raw, ripe organic fruits and veggies (real 'fast food' with high water content) in your diet. Beverages or fluids that contain caffeine or other stimulants, refined sugar, refined salt*, artificial sweeteners, and synthetic vitamins and minerals can cause dehydration. Many drugs, chemicals and personal care products can also rob the body of water and may increase your water needs as well. So, maintaining proper hydration is about more than just consuming enough water; it's also about NOT consuming items that pull water out of your body!

*__Note:__ *In general, refined salt is dehydrating, so limiting it in your diet may be wise. The body does need sodium to function correctly, which can be found in many natural foods, especially fruits and veggies and other produce. However, refined salt (a mineral compound called sodium chloride) shouldn't be confused with sodium.*

Feeling thirsty may not always be a reliable sign that your body needs more water, as this signal can become blunted if you're already dehydrated. Thirst is an instinct, but like many other human instincts, it can become diminished over time, especially if the body has been neglected or abused. Other signs of dehydration (besides thirst) include lethargy and fatigue; mental confusion; absence of sweating in spite of heavy activity; decreased physical and/or mental performance; sunken eyes; absence of tears when crying vigorously; dry mouth; chills; nausea; perceived hunger*; cramps; restless or irritable behavior; weak rapid pulse; flushed face; dry or warm skin; very little urine output; urine that is strong smelling and dark yellow in appearance; dizziness; weakness; headaches; and pain (especially in an injured region of the body).

*Note: Many times, 'perceived hunger' is really the body's cry for more water. So, if you think you're hungry but not sure, then have some water first and see what happens. Hunger will persist if food is what your body really wants.

Paying attention to your body's warning signs of dehydration is important. When really dehydrated, your sense of thirst will actually return after consuming some water, indicating that you need to drink even more water. Your urine should be pale yellow to clear in appearance when hydrated correctly. (Note: Vitamin supplements and/or some medications can sometimes change the color of urine). By the way, you should be peeing several times a day if healthy (up to six to ten times), so you should have plenty of chances throughout the day to keep track of your urine color. Using a scale to measure your body weight before and after exercise or activity can also be an effective tool to help measure water loss and prevent dehydration.

Sources Of Water

There's water in most beverages, so some of your water needs will be met if you consume them. Again, just be mindful that whatever you're consuming isn't a 'water robber', so as not to dehydrate yourself. I would recommend avoiding most commercial beverages including alcohol, dairy products, caffeinated beverages, energy drinks, sports drinks, carbonated drinks, soda, and pasteurized juices. Beverages recommended besides good clean water would include fresh-squeezed fruit and veggie juices or smoothies, and coconut water. Some non-caffeinated herbal teas, or fruit and spice teas may be okay as well. Eating and drinking isn't the only way your body absorbs water. Water absorption can also occur through the skin. So, the water you bathe in should also be a consideration. This is a good reason to consider buying a water filtration system for your house.

What Kind Of Water Is Best?

It's important that you consume (drink, as well as bathe in) clean water. Therefore, I would recommend that your water be filtered in a way that removes most of the chemicals (such as chlorine and fluoride), bacteria and micro-organisms, heavy metals, pesticides, radiation, etc. There are various filtration systems on the market that can serve this purpose (even water bottles that can filter water). Bottom line: Most tap water is very polluted, and most bottled water often is as well. Just remember: *If you don't use a filter, your body may become the filter!*

*Bonus: Learn what questions you should consider before buying a water filtration system. Visit: FeelGoodNowTheBook.com. Enter bonus code: FGN8

How To Drink

All liquids (including water) should be sipped, not gulped. They should also be mixed adequately with your saliva before swallowing. Mixing your beverages (as well as food) with your saliva signals to your body what is entering, so that your body can be properly prepared to utilize it. Your mouth is the gatekeeper to the rest of your digestive system. It contains substances (immune cells and enzymes) that can help to ensure the neutralization and/or destruction of anything undesirable (bacteria or toxins, for example) that may be trying to enter the body. Swishing the beverages around in your mouth thoroughly before you swallow them can help to ensure they're mixed with your saliva. (No, you don't have to gargle it too!)

Drinking extremely hot or cold water (or other beverages), especially quickly, is not recommended as this can be traumatic to your insides. Bottom line: If you can't hold a liquid in your mouth comfortably, then you shouldn't swallow it. It's also wise to avoid drinking large amounts of water (or other fluids) along with your meals because this can dilute your digestive juices and can impair digestion. If whatever you're eating is making you thirsty, it's highly questionable whether or not you should be eating much of that food in the first place. Lastly, just like eating, make sure to drink out of necessity, not habit. If you don't need water, then don't force it down. Again, the whole point of being properly hydrated is to help you feel good now, not turn yourself into an aquarium!

The following 'Link Builder' will help you address your 'Water Link' when it needs attention. Reading or saying this phrase often can serve as a nice reminder about the importance of staying well hydrated to feel good now!

Link Builder: **Feeling down and out may be due to drought— consume more water!**

Chapter 6

Link #4- Light
Are You 'Scared' Of The Light?

Natural light is very important to your health. What is the main source of light on this planet? That big bright fire ball in the sky called the sun. Sunlight is more than just a bright light though. It's part of an electromagnetic spectrum consisting of over twelve hundred frequencies of light that have key benefits to the body. Each wavelength may have a specific role to play in your health. Sunlight helps to power your cells, regulate your biological clock (circadian rhythms) and help you produce hormones. When you're not getting enough sunlight, health can start to decline quickly. Sunshine is the best source of Vitamin D for the body; a vitamin that is imperative for the prevention of many types of cancer (including skin cancer).

For many people, lack of natural light during the winter months is a common reason for low energy and depression. You need sunlight on an ongoing basis to remain healthy. Natural light is probably one of the most under-rated nutrients that belongs in one's diet. Have you ever noticed how you feel when the sun isn't shining? Not so good, huh? How about when the sun breaks through on a cloudy day? Yes, it's like an instant shot of 'feel good now', isn't it? Let there be light!

How Much Sun?

Just like water, one's sun requirements can change from day to day, so it's important to, once again, listen to your body and give it what it needs. With that being said, you should get *enough* sun each day. In other words, once you have received all the sun that is needed, get out of the sun. For some reason, every other species seems to do this correctly except us humans. Sunbathing with little clothing (or sometimes with no clothing at all) is preferable to get the maximum health benefits from the sun. If nude sunbathing is not permissible where you live, then you could wear a 'tan through' bathing suit. These suits allow the sun in, but not other people's eyes.

Sun exposure through glass windows is not the same as direct sun exposure. More benefits from the sun will occur with direct sun. Surfaces such as sand, snow, concrete, and water can reflect a large amount of the ultraviolet radiation. Therefore, extra precautions should be taken when around these surfaces to avoid overexposure. The further from the equator you live, and the darker your skin color, the more sun you may need to feel good and remain healthy. Fair-skinned people usually need less sun. People with more body fat will usually need more sunshine.

There are essentially three main types of ultraviolet light: A, B and C. Types A and B are considered the more essential ones. Overall, tanning is desirable, but burning is not (so pay attention to your body). There are two very common recommendations often given about sun protection that deserve reconsideration. The first is to wear sunblocks and lotions. Unfortunately, most of these products often contain chemicals that are either skin irritants or carcinogens (cause cancer). Kind of ironic, huh? Aren't these products supposed to have the opposite effect? If you do decide to wear any form of commercial sunblocks, then please do some research first and know exactly what you're rubbing on your skin!

The second recommendation is to avoid the mid-day hours of the sun. However, these are the same hours when UVB rays are the highest (UVB rays help your body produce Vitamin D). So, if many people have been following these two common recommendations for awhile, is it really any wonder why there's a current epidemic of Vitamin D deficiency and cancer going on? Sunbathing with chlorine (from the pool) on your skin is not recommended either, as this can lead to burning and skin irritation. This should be common sense, but people do it all the time.

*Bonus: Learn some of the best types of natural sunscreen that you can wear. Visit: FeelGoodNowTheBook.com. Enter bonus code: FGN8

"Keep your face always towards the sunshine-and shadows will fall behind you."
-Walt Whitman

Light Phobia

People have become so 'sun phobic' these days, it's ridiculous. One should be more afraid of artificial light, as opposed to fearing natural sunlight. Consuming large amounts of artificial light (mal-illumination) may be considered a form of malnutrition—and it can definitely lead to that very same condition as well! Fluorescent lighting is not recommended, as it's a form of radiation that isn't healthy for the body. If you work or live under this type of lighting all the time, then you may have become accustomed to it and not noticed it's damaging effects upon your health. However, being accustomed to something doesn't mean that you are immune to it. People become accustomed to all kinds of things that still impact their health in a negative manner (smoking, alcohol, drugs, chemicals, for example).

Mal-illumination = Malnutrition = Not Feeling Good!

or

Poor Lighting = Poor Nourishment = Poor Health!

Light Bulbs

Many types of artificial lights, such as incandescent bulbs (ordinary light bulbs), fluorescent lights, sodium lights, and halogens all produce a yellow frequency. Too much yellow puts a strain on the eye, which is why these bulbs may make you squint when using them (a sign they're probably not good for us), especially when reading. The incandescent bulb was developed because its bright yellow color reached the eyes quickly. However, this yellow light can cause your eyes (and your body) to contract when you're exposed to it. This places your body under constant stress, which leads to poor health.

Although commonly used, fluorescent lights should be avoided if possible. Besides emitting a color frequency that isn't optimal for eye function, some fluorescents also flicker as well as emit a type of radiation (equivalent to a soft x-ray) from the ends of the tubes. This can cause difficulty concentrating as well as places continual negative stress on your body that jeopardizes your health. Compact fluorescents became popular for their 'energy efficiency' qualities. Although they may save one some money from the electric company, they may cost a great amount of money when it comes to having better health. Besides the poor qualities of fluorescents already mentioned, compact fluorescent lights (aka 'CFL's') do contain mercury—a toxic heavy metal that has been linked to many serious health conditions. The fact that there's a 'hazardous material protocol' that's recommended if you were to break one of these lights in your home should say enough!

How will you know if fluorescent lighting really bothers you? The answer is simple: You're going to have to be the scientist, use your body as the laboratory, run the experiment, collect the data, and then apply what you've learned. Okay, that didn't sound very simple, did it? However, it really is. For example, if you want to determine if fluorescent lighting is negatively impacting your health, then you need to spend some quality time away from it (all day long) for at least two weeks. Take note of how you feel. Then, start to expose yourself to fluorescent lighting again all day long and note any differences in how you feel. You may be surprised at what you discover: more energy, better focus and concentration, better sleep, better mood, better appearance, better sex (seriously)...and the list could go on!

Full-Spectrum Lighting

If you choose to live in a region of the world where there's less than optimal sun light, or you just want to feel better overall, then using 'full-spectrum lights' may help. 'Full-spectrum light' refers to a light source that covers the entire range of visible light without having any gaps in its spectrum output. These lights emit white light that has little to no glare at all (which is why one can often read for hours under these lights without

38

squinting or feeling eyestrain). It may take approximately six hours of 'full-spectrum lighting' exposure to be equivalent to thirty minutes of natural sunlight. This is good news if you work in an office, since you have to be there all day long anyway. If you're going to buy 'full-spectrum lights', then just make sure to ask questions so you're getting the real thing. True 'full-spectrum lights' will usually have a Kelvin temperature range of five thousand to fifty-nine hundred and a CRI (Color Rendering Index) of about ninety or above.) Many of the bulbs that claim to be full-spectrum aren't always the real deal. A true full-spectrum bulb contains a good amount of ultraviolet light. There are some bulbs on the market also called 'total spectrum bulbs' or 'extra-brights', which have some ultraviolet in them (and may be beneficial as well).

Although replacing your fluorescents with full-spectrum bulbs can definitely be a 'quick fix' to feeling better, are 'full-spectrum lights' a good substitute for natural sunlight? Of course not; but they're a good substitute for other poor lighting schemes. The best option is to find a way to allow more natural light to come into your home or work environment whenever possible.

Nature's Master Rhythm

Natural light helps to regulate the body's internal clock, aid in hormone production and help produce the energy that goes to your cells so they can function properly. Therefore, it would be wise to obey 'Nature's Master Rhythm'—the sun-cycle—meaning you're up when the sun's up and down when the sun's down. If you violate this rule on a consistent basis, your health may suffer and you'll never know how good you could possibly feel. You may be saying to yourself right now, "But, I'm a night-owl!" Being a 'night-owl' (a person who stays up late at night) is a learned behavior. We're not nocturnal creatures by nature.

If you appear to get a 'second wind' at night, it's usually because you've put your body into a stress mode and over-stimulated it, which often leads to a feeling of more alertness. Although you may desire this, your body doesn't—so keep the lights off at night! How will you know if this is really true? Again, you'll have to run an experiment. Keep the lights low (better yet, most of them off) at night and see if you still 'feel awake' and have the desire to stay up late. By the way, if you have hormonal imbalances, it would benefit you to keep the lights low and to get to bed early. Again, light plays a vital role in regulating hormones.

The following 'Link Builder' will help you address your 'Light Link' when it needs attention. Reading or saying this phrase often can serve as a nice reminder about the importance of natural light to feel good now!

Link Builder: **Natural light by day is the feel good way. Artificial light by night can cause strife!**

Chapter 7

Link #5- Rest
A 'Reliable' Method For Improving How You Feel!

When it comes to feeling better, rest is one of the best remedies known to mankind. I've developed a simple mnemonic for the word rest. R.E.S.T. = Reliable Easy Safe Technique. Rest helps recharge your batteries every day. It's at rest, when your body heals best. It's at rest, when your body and mind can integrate. It's at rest, when spiritual enlightenment will often occur. It's at rest, when your body performs its miraculous wonders of repair and cleansing (detoxification). When your body is allowed to rest, a vital power reserve can be built up and stored, which can then later be used to meet the demands placed upon it. Rest is part of nature's master plan of health and of life.

There are many ways to secure rest. Mental-emotional rest can be achieved when one quiets the mind of internal chatter or noise and finds a place of peace. Meditation can bring about such a state. Physiological rest occurs when sleeping and fasting (not eating). Sensory rest may be achieved by closing one's eyes, ears, nose, mouth, and/or abstaining from touching or being touched, and thus taking a break from using the senses to interact with the environment. Physical rest occurs when sleeping, napping, or just resting the body in a comfortable position. All forms of rest are necessary for good health.

Stimulants

Living on stimulants (such as caffeine, nicotine, energy drinks) is a mistake. It may provide the body with a short-term high, but this will always be followed by a long-term low. Even though caffeine is 'all-natural', it doesn't mean it's really safe. Stimulants don't give you energy; they just over-stimulate your nervous system, which only leads to further exhausting your body and making you more tired. It's kind of like whipping a tired horse. If you do this, in the short-run the horse may perform okay, but eventually the horse's performance will suffer in the

41

long-run. If the horse is tired, give him rest. The same goes for you—always rest when needed.

Just like a car, you have a battery and a gas tank. Would you ever try to recharge your battery by filling your gas tank? Why not? It's not logical; and it wouldn't work! Well, the body is no different. If your battery (nervous system) is drained, trying to recharge it by filling your gas tank (stomach), especially with the wrong kind of fuel (stimulants like caffeine or junk food) won't work! Rest is nature's true caffeine. When your body is thoroughly rested, you will have all the energy you ever need. Speaking of cars, if you need to drive but are tired, then pull over and rest for a bit. Driving tired or strung out on stimulants is not healthy or safe. There is a reason places along the highways are called 'rest stops' (use them wisely). If there are none available, then find another safe, quiet place that you can park for a bit to give your body the rest it needs to feel good and stay well.

"A good laugh and a long sleep are the best cures in the doctor's book."
-Irish Proverb

How Much Sleep?

Like other health needs (such as food, water and light), one needs *enough* sleep each day. Therefore, your sleep requirements will vary depending on the demands being placed upon your body. Generally speaking, if you need an alarm clock to wake up in the morning, you're not getting enough sleep. By the way, why would you want to start each day stressed and 'alarmed'? This just isn't healthy. You should wake up naturally on a daily basis feeling revitalized and ready to move (without an alarm clock). If this isn't the case, you're sleep deprived. If you're using stimulants (such as caffeine, herbs, or drugs) to constantly boost your energy levels, then more sleep is needed. Remember, health is earned. So, if a 'sleep debt' has been accumulated, it must be repaid. Otherwise, your body will not function or feel well. To repay a sleep debt, you should go to bed an hour (or more) earlier each night until you're caught up on sleep.

Napping for ten to twenty minutes in the middle of the day can help to repay a sleep debt as well. Many people have become conditioned to believe that taking a nap in the middle of the day or just lying down and resting for ten to fifteen minutes is a big waste of time, as they have 'better things to do'. Well, if not properly rested, it will be hard to accomplish these other things. Feeling tired is a result of getting too little sleep (especially deep stages of sleep), not a result of getting too much sleep, which is really hard to do.

In times of increased stress (injury or illness, for example), your body will require more rest and sleep. Neglecting to make this accommodation at such times can delay healing and prolong the recovery process. No doubt, rest and sleep are some of the best known remedies available to us. There is no substitute for rest when needed. Reaching for a pillow (instead of some pills) may be the wiser choice when you really want to heal and feel better quickly!

Quality Of Rest Is Important

Getting to bed on the earlier side each night is wise. As mentioned in the last chapter, there really is no such thing as a 'night owl' (a person who likes to stay up late). Again, this is a learned behavior; as well as a bad habit. Although you might feel good at the time, this is not how to achieve the 'feel good now' theme of this book as you won't be building better health with this late-night habit. If you think that you're a night owl, then I encourage you to run this simple experiment: Keep the main lights off in your house at night and see what happens. Yes, you'll go 'nighty night' pretty quickly! Don't fight this urge to go to sleep. Yes, you may wake up earlier if you go to bed earlier. That's the whole point. As mentioned previously (see Chapter 6), by following the light-dark cycles, your body will become more in tune with 'Natures Master Rhythm', which helps to regulate and ensure optimal health.

What you do once in awhile won't matter as much as what you do on a consistent basis. So, if you have to be up late now and then, it's probably not a big deal. However, if you're going to be up late, try to minimize the lighting you need and don't eat late either. As a general guideline, avoid eating just prior to going to bed (at least two hours), especially consuming any stimulants, such as caffeine, nicotine, or junk foods.

The better you take care of yourself during the day, the better you'll sleep at night. If you suffer with insomnia (difficulty sleeping), this doesn't need to keep happening. Insomnia can be caused by an over-stimulated nervous system brought on by unhealthful diet and lifestyle habits. So, if you choose to abuse your body (either intentionally or unintentionally) during the day, then there's a price to pay—your body will keep you up at night! Your body has to maintain balance (homeostasis) in order to remain healthy. The harder it has to work at night to maintain this balance, the more difficult it may be for you to sleep.

Sleep Should Help You Recover

You shouldn't have to recover from sleep; your sleep should help you recover! Therefore, if you want better sleep, then your sleeping environment needs to be conducive to providing you with better sleep. You're a product of your environment—sleep being no exception to this rule. Both your internal (your body) and external (place where you sleep) environments matter. Would you like a twelve-point checklist for better sleep? Yes? Here you go:

Twelve-point Checklist for Better Sleep

1. Keep your sleeping environment quiet and well ventilated.
2. Going to bed well hydrated will help you sleep better.
3. Go to bed on an empty stomach (stop eating at least two hours prior to bed). Just remember: If your body is too busy digesting, it won't be resting!
4. Keep your sleeping environment dark (minimize any lighting) and a comfortable temperature (cooler is often better).
5. Get to bed by 10pm at the latest (9pm would be better). When you sleep is just as important as how much time you sleep. Therefore, sleep quality is just as important as quantity. The body's natural

44

circadian rhythms should be respected. If you miss the key hours of sleep each night, you will not feel as good. Remember to obey 'Nature's Master Rhythm'.

6. Avoid engaging in stimulating activities (exercise, reading, TV, for example) just prior to bed that may prevent you from relaxing and falling asleep.

7. Keep your sleeping environment free of EMF's (electromagnetic fields) as they can disrupt your quality of sleep. This means keep all electrical appliances (TV, radio, clocks, phones, etc.) out of your sleeping area to help reduce any EMF stress. Positioning your bed in the middle of the room (as opposed to against a wall) can also help minimize EMF stress as this will keep the wiring in your walls further away from your head. You should also shut off your wireless router (WiFi) at night to minimize stress to your body while trying to sleep.

8. Getting plenty of exercise, sunshine, fresh air, wholesome foods, and water during the day will help you sleep better at night.

9. Go to bed with love in your heart. If you're angry or upset in any way, deal with your feelings and then let them go. Stop worrying. If something is on your mind, write it down so you can put your mind and body at rest.

10. Keep a consistent sleep schedule. Go to bed around the same time.

11. Sleeping slightly inverted (so your feet are higher than your head) may help to promote very rejuvenating sleep.

12. Your bedding should consist of natural, organic materials that allows your body to breathe. Whatever you clean your bedding and linens with should also not cause you any bodily distress. Your bed should make you well and rested, not sick and tired.

Take A 'Time-Out' And Reboot!

When kids misbehave, they may be put in a 'time-out'. This usually involves removing children from the environment they're in and placing them in a quiet place where they can calm down and reflect a bit. When done correctly, this can be a valuable tool to help a child connect his actions and behaviors with how they feel. It also provides the child with a stress coping mechanism and a way to deal with life's situations. Guess what? Adults may continue to benefit from going into a 'time out' as well. Why? Adults misbehave and get stressed also. So, when feeling ill, frazzled, unsure, or overwhelmed, just take a 'time out' and allow yourself a chance to rest and reflect.

As simple as taking a 'time out' sounds, so many people don't do it. They keep pushing on and get more stressed out instead (which leads to the opposite of feeling good now). If you don't like the concept of a 'time out', then how about 'take a break'? If you don't take a break when needed, you may definitely end up feeling 'broken' for sure. It really doesn't matter what you call it. You just have to do it! Even something as simple as just closing your eyes for at least ten seconds a few times an hour (especially when working on a computer) can help you feel less frazzled and more refreshed. When a computer is not working correctly, taking the time to reboot it will often correct the problem. Give your body the same love and care by rebooting each day as needed.

Bonus: Learn a simple exercise to help you reboot your body each day. Visit: FeelGoodNowTheBook.com. Enter bonus code: FGN8

The following 'Link Builder' will help you address your 'Rest Link' when it needs attention. Reading or saying this phrase often can serve as a nice reminder about the importance of staying well rested to feel good now!

Link Builder: **If you want to feel your best, then take some R.E.S.T.!**

Chapter 8

Link #6- Activity
You Must 'Move Well' To Feel Well!

In the last chapter, you learned the importance of resting. In this chapter, you'll learn that it's also important to move! There are definitely way too many 'sit-downs' being done these days around the world. 'Sit-downs' are where a person sits down on their buttocks for most of the day and doesn't move very much. This isn't conducive to good health. You need to move. Life depends on movement. Without such movement (physical activity/exercise), your body will be prone to weakness, degeneration, and poor health!

Healthy bodies move, look, feel and sound good. They don't jerk, limp, creak, crackle and pop, or have a funny shape; nor are they stiff, painful, obese, irritable, depressed, or stressed. Yes, movement can help you feel better, look better, and function better overall. This means you'll be more fit and beautiful, have more energy, be in a better mood, think better, sleep better, digest better, eliminate better, have better sex; and just be a better person. Does this sound like something you desire?

"Lack of activity destroys the good condition of every human being, while movement and methodical physical exercise save it and preserve it." -Plato

How Much Activity?

How much should you move and exercise each day? Just like many of the other links in the Chain-of-Health System™, the answer is: *enough*. The amount should always be proportionate to the body's needs at any given time. For example, during rehabilitation from an injury, too much or too little movement can impair the body's ability to heal and repair itself correctly. When not injured, too much exercise can lead to injury; whereas not enough may also lead to a body prone to injury as well. Overall, exercise shouldn't be injurious to your body. This means that exercise isn't supposed to hurt you. Somewhere along the way though, you have been told that if exercise doesn't make you sore, then it's not beneficial. You have been told, "No pain, no gain!" Unfortunately, this philosophy gets many people in big trouble.

If the kind of movement or exercise that you're performing hurts, then you should probably stop doing it. This should be common sense. There may be a number of reasons why an exercise may be causing pain. The important point to understand is that despite the cause, you should listen to your body's pain signals and obey them. Since your body has to adapt to the physical demands placed upon it, you may become a bit sore after performing an activity that you're not used to. This is okay. (If you can't walk the next day, this is NOT okay!). You may also feel some brief discomfort when a beneficial change is occurring while exercising (when scar tissue releases, for example). P.A.I.N. (Pay Attention Important Now) is one of the ways your body intelligently protects itself. When an activity hurts, you should pay attention and either modify the activity so it doesn't hurt, or just stop doing it completely!

__Bonus:__ Learn the reasons why you might have pain while exercising. Visit: FeelGoodNowTheBook.com. Enter bonus code: FGN8

Although exercise should make you feel better, it's important that these feelings of well-being are a result of the exercise benefiting you, not over-stimulating you. In other words, exercise shouldn't be like a drug that you become addicted to! Just like eating, if you abuse exercise (do too much or do the wrong kinds), your body will not be nourished correctly. Although you may feel good initially after exercising incorrectly (due to the adrenal rush and 'pick-me-up' you get), the rebound effect will not be a pleasant one as you come down, and your health will eventually suffer if you continue this habit.

If exercising too much, you may eventually end up irritable; restless; having difficulty sleeping; moody; fatigued; having nagging pains; feeling ill, having decreased appetite; experiencing decreased motivation; having decreased libido; demonstrating decreased athletic performance; or not recovering well from your previous workout. Pay attention for these signs. If they appear, then cut back on the amount of activity that you're doing and allow your body to recover. The point of exercise is to *train and gain,* not *strain and drain* your body.

What Kind Of Exercise?

What kind of exercise or movement is best? The answer is: It depends. Overall, I think doing the kind of exercise that you enjoy, that's safe, and that's conducive to building and maintaining good health is the best kind. If an exercise doesn't promote, enhance or maintain your health and function, then is it really worth doing at all? If you have specific postural deformities, joint or orthopedic problems, chronic aches and pains, muscle imbalances, or poor movement patterns, then I would recommend consulting a qualified health or fitness practitioner (such as a physical therapist, chiropractor, strength and conditioning coach, or corrective exercise specialist) to get those issues corrected with a customized exercise program that is designed specifically for you.

Remember, a chain is only as strong as its weakest link. Your body's 'kinetic chain' (muscles, bones, nerves, connective tissues) is only as strong as its weakest link also. For example, if you have a stiff ankle because of a misalignment in the bones of your foot, you'll always be limited by this weak link. Exercising incorrectly with this ankle dysfunction will usually only reinforce it, not correct it. It may even cause other problems eventually, as your body will learn to compensate in other regions to take stress off the stiff ankle region. Trying to build or maintain fitness on top of an existing problem is not wise or advised. It's like trying to drive a car around with a flat tire hoping the tire will somehow just fix itself. It just isn't going to happen! Bottom line: *Quality of movement is just as important as quantity of movement.* If you don't move well, then you can't exercise well. Again, if you need to find a good coach, trainer or therapist to help you get back into better shape, then do it.

Gyms

You don't need a gym to exercise. You can exercise anywhere. Gyms are often just an excuse for most people to avoid exercising. It sounds something like this: 'I don't have time to go the gym.' or 'The gym is not open.' or 'The gym is too far away.' or 'The gym is (fill in the blank)'...you get the point! My favorite gym is 'Mother Nature's Gym'. Where is this located? Just about everywhere you look outside. One place I love to exercise is in my garden and orchard. I like to call this 'envirocise', which is exercise that benefits both you and the environment. When you think about it, if you're going to spend the time moving around or engaged in hard labor, why not get an extra benefit (food) from doing it? Besides, most people spend way too much time indoors anyway. Go outside and exercise. This will allow you to get some fresh air and sunshine as well (which were some of those other important health links discussed in earlier chapters).

Lastly, your body is the gym! You don't need fancy equipment or things that light up, beep, or tell you how many calories you've burned. All you need is a little motivation and some creativity. I've exercised everywhere—on planes, subways, trains, cars, beaches, houses, playgrounds, parking lots...and the list goes on. There really are no limits to where you can exercise with just using your own bodyweight. Gymnasts often use bodyweight exercise as a primary part of their training for a good reason; it builds not only size and strength, but also overall athleticism. You don't have to turn yourself into a gymnast, but including bodyweight exercise in your fitness regimen can be very beneficial to your health, as well as to your survival!

Work And Hobbies

Besides exercise, work and hobbies also count as activity (that is, if you actually move around while performing them). If your work or hobbies require a heavy amount of manual labor, then you may not need to perform as much exercise in order to remain healthy. Just so we're clear, moving a mouse around on a desk all day while at the computer, or playing checkers or cards, is not heavy manual labor. What I'm talking about is the type of job that requires frequent lifting, squatting, bending, pushing, pulling, climbing steps or ladders, digging, etc., several days a week. When this is the case, it would be wise to perform some different types of movements or activities that are less intense and allow your body to move in a different manner than it has been moving. For example, if you have been squatting all day long, then engaging in some form of physical activity or exercise that doesn't require squatting would be a good choice (such as walking). This will help keep your body's structure (posture and alignment) better balanced and prevent you from overusing certain parts and injuring yourself. If your work is long and intense, then your exercise or leisure activities should be far less in intensity and duration.

Fitness For Health

In order to be healthy, you must be a fit person. In order to be a fit person, you must be an active person—you must move! There really are no days off when it comes to fitness. This doesn't mean you should be exercising or engaging in intense physical activities constantly. What it means is that every day you can be doing something to improve and/or maintain your level of fitness. If you spend just even ten to fifteen minutes a day dedicated to some fitness activity, it can help you significantly improve your health and feel good now! Fitness is a lifestyle habit. Like most other habits, if you develop the 'habit of fitness', it will be hard to break and you will become committed to it.

At a minimum, just walking one to two miles each day can help keep you feeling good. When should you go for a walk? Anytime would be fine. However, each day your body will 'talk' to you, and there will be an urge to move (you might feel stiff or a bit 'antsy', for example). So, pay attention. When your body starts to talk, just move or take a walk! Personally, I like to walk a few times a day, especially in the morning. A nice leisurely walk outside is a great way to get moving, connect with nature, and become better prepared for the rest of the day.

51

The following 'Link Builder' will help you address your 'Activity Link' when it needs attention. Reading or saying this phrase often can serve as a nice reminder about the importance of exercising to feel good now!

Link Builder: **When your body starts to talk, it's time to move or take a walk!**

Chapter 9

Link #7- Hygiene
'Let Go' To Stay In The 'Feel Good Now' Flow!

When it comes to feeling better, there's no doubt that good hygiene is important. You're a product of your environment, both inside and out. Therefore, keeping your body (as well as your living environment) clean is an important part of the 'feel good now' health equation. One of the best ways to keep your body clean is to avoid polluting it in the first place. This has been emphasized in earlier chapters. Although it's important to pay attention to what goes into your body, it's also important to pay attention when something needs to come out.

Your body is a self-cleansing organism. This means that it will secrete certain body fluids and/or attempt to eliminate irritants and wastes on a daily basis. When the body is intelligently carrying out this act of survival, it's best to assist (rather than interfere with) this process. For example, mucus discharge is a cleansing process. It shouldn't be suppressed, but rather allowed to come out instead. This is called 'cleansing'. If you want the mucus discharge to stop, then remove the cause of why it's there to begin with and it will go away.

Ironically, many people in the 'cleaning industry' often suffer from sniffles and mucus discharge because of the irritating cleaning products they're constantly using. You would think that eventually they would figure it out. However, if they're around these harsh cleaners all the time, they probably can't make the connection between them and the reason for their suffering (runny nose, itchy watery eyes, or coughing and sneezing fits). There are two lessons here: First, if your body is being irritated, it will give you clear and definite signs so pay attention. Second, when you're cleaning something, don't pollute your body or the environment around you.

"Hygiene is two thirds of health."
-Lebanese Proverb

Germs

Ever since the invention of modern day so-called 'antibacterial' soaps and lotions, it seems that we're sicker than ever. Why might this be? Well, the skin contains its own bacteria that are important for protecting the body from foreign invaders. If this protective layer of bacteria is constantly under attack, then it doesn't work too well. Germs aren't usually the primary causes of most poor health conditions. Many germs occasion a health problem, but they don't cause it. This means that although they're often found at the crime scene, they didn't commit the crime. In other words, the germs are actually there to help out, but they often get erroneously blamed for causing the problem. They're often then punished for trying to lend a hand (attacked or killed with drugs, chemicals, etc.). This approach often does not work too well, which is becoming more apparent these days as seen by the increasing number of resistant strains of germs that are developing.

Germs have a vital role to play in life, and it's often a symbiotic one. Many germs are scavengers. Their job is to clean up garbage or debris that needs to be discarded. So, most of the time, they are your friends, not your enemies. There are always tons of germs in, on, and around your body all the time. There are many more times the number of germs in your body than there are cells. This should be an important clue as to their significance as it pertains to your health. You need germs in order to function properly. If they were the true cause of most health problems, we would all be long dead by now!

So, what's the best way to keep germs in a healthy balance and working for you, not against you? The key is the terrain (or environment). It's the terrain that causes the germ, not really the other way around. The following analogy may help you understand this concept better. Flies don't cause garbage; it's the other way around. The flies are there because there is garbage there to feed on. Remove the garbage, and the flies will go away. Likewise, removing the garbage (junk food, chemicals, drugs, radiation, toxins) from your body, home, and working environments, as well as not putting garbage in there to begin with, will help the undesirable germs go away. Again, most germs are beneficial; and the undesirable ones are best dealt with by establishing a healthy terrain (using good hygiene and healthy lifestyle habits) to become an intolerable host—as opposed to trying to kill the germs using toxic chemicals. When caring for your body, learn to cooperate with nature, not fight it. Let's end the 'war on terra', shall we?

Detoxification

'Detoxification' has become a huge buzz word in the last several years. Many people seem to be on 'detox diets' and 'detox programs'. However, there seems to be much confusion and debate on how best to detoxify the body. To keep this matter simple, let's consider some basic things about detox. First, detoxification is an ongoing process that never ends. Your body has to be able to deal with wastes that accumulate. The good news is that your body is built to detoxify itself. Just think about its design. Some of your largest organs (liver, lungs, kidneys, stomach, spleen, intestines, and skin) are detox organs. This means that in order to detoxify your body correctly, you need to treat it correctly (by following the Chain-of-Health System™). Don't waste large amounts of time, money and energy with expensive, complicated 'detox products' that are often unnecessary, unsafe, and ineffective. (Reminder: Health is earned!)

Bonus: Learn why being barefoot may actually be a 'clean' thing to do. Visit: FeelGoodNowTheBook.com. Enter bonus code: FGN8

Taking Care Of Business

If you do find the need to 'take something' to help detoxify your body to feel better, then definitely make it a habit to *take the time* to allow your body to do its thing when needed. For example, when you have to go to the bathroom, then go. There are times when your 'Number Two' business needs to become your number one business (so take care of it). It's amazing to me that people will suppress the urge to void (poop) for minutes, hours, or even days on end! Worse yet, they then take a bunch of detox potions and pills, or put a hose up their butt to try and get a 'quick fix'. In case you need a reminder: Having a couple of bowel movements every day is normal. Yes, that's right. You are supposed to poop every day; and at least one to two feet of it should be coming out of you as well. As unbelievable as that may sound, that is normal (just not common) bowel health.

When you do have to go, then you should assume the correct voiding position, which is a deep squat. This may be much easier to do when out in nature versus when using an inside standard bathroom. (When inside, I personally assume the deep squat position on top of the toilet. Yes, I've had a few almost fall-in-the-toilet moments, so be sure to check that the toilet—both the seat, as well as the toilet itself—is safe and sturdy before you attempt this.) If you can't squat down deeply, then placing your feet on a small stool so that the knees are above your hips while sitting on the toilet may also help. This places the body in a position that allows your bowels to empty themselves out better. Whether you're an adult or child, sitting on the potty with your legs dangling and feet off the floor is not conducive to performing a bowel movement efficiently. This means that you will retain more toxins, which leads to not feeling good now!

As for 'Number One' (urinating, peeing, wee-wee, tinkle, whiz or whatever else you want to call it), the same main rule applies: When you have to go, then go! No, it's not an 'inconvenience'; it's your body's way of helping you remain healthy and feeling good. Urinating several times a day is normal by the way. If you think this is inconvenient, try having bladder, rectal, or urogenital pain or cancer. You don't have to squat down to urinate correctly, but you can if you want to. (Ladies, I think most of you already do this. Fellas, just be careful and make sure there's plenty of clearance and no sharp objects in the way first.)

Voiding (pooping and peeing) is an act of survival. Without it, the body will not function properly. Therefore, this instinct of self-preservation shouldn't be suppressed. It's always sad to hear when a child is denied permission to use the bathroom and made to 'hold it', especially when there's no good reason to do so. What does this really accomplish? Not much, other than making a child self-conscious about a natural act that helps to keep him/her well. If this bad habit ('holding it') is carried into adulthood, it can definitely lead to poor health as the body's sanitation department is not being allowed to do its job correctly.

Other Stuff

There are various other ways that the body will rid itself of something that isn't needed. It may do this via: coughing, sneezing, throwing up, discharging (mucus removal from nose, ears, mouth or other bodily orifices), bleeding (such as menses), gas removal (burping or farting), or by sweating. All of these are a purging process and shouldn't be suppressed. You may not feel good doing some of them during the process, but you'll usually feel better quickly afterwards. Don't be embarrassed. Be happy your body is working correctly instead. So, if there really isn't a good reason that you can't let it go, then let it go. In other words: When Nature calls, be sure to answer! Others will understand; but at the same time, always be respectful of those around you before you do answer the call of duty! (Yes, pun intended.)

Keeping The Outside Clean

Make sure to keep track of your external living space. This includes your house, car, boat, office and any other places that you may occupy on a regular basis as well. Keep them all clean. This may seem like a big chore, but trust me, it's nothing compared with the chore of being sick all the time. If you clean as you go and don't let things pile up, this won't seem like such a daunting task. If you do feel overwhelmed with cleaning, then just ask for help. Either get some family or friends to help out (you may have to bribe them), or hire somebody to help you get the job done right. Just make sure that whoever you hire will use natural (non-toxic) cleaning methods to avoid polluting your living space. As mentioned earlier (see Chapter 4), many people often pollute the very air they breathe. Just as harsh chemicals don't clean the air, they also don't clean your living space well either (at least not without jeopardizing your health).

Clutter creates chaos. If you want to test this, just stand in a room that is neat and orderly and note how you feel. Then, compare this experience with how you feel when you're in a messy and cluttered space. There usually is a noticeable difference. You can become accustomed to your own clutter to the point that you don't even notice it anymore. If you're unsure whether or not you have too much clutter around you, then just ask others (who'll be honest with you). Do you need to be a 'Feng Shui Master' to have better health? No, but paying a bit more attention to keeping the space around you both clean and organized may help you feel much better.

The following 'Link Builder' will help you address your 'Hygiene Link' when it needs attention. Reading or saying this phrase often can serve as a nice reminder about the importance of good hygiene to feel good now!

Link Builder: **If you want your health to beam, then you must keep your body and living space clean!**

Chapter 10

Link #8- Love
The 'Master Link' For Better Health!

Within a chain, there's often a 'master-link'. In one's Chain-of-Health System™, the master link would be love. Without love (especially self-love), the other links will always be weak. Why? You have to love yourself enough to eat well, drink and bathe in clean water, take in fresh air and breathe correctly, get enough rest and sleep, consume adequate sunshine, exercise regularly, and maintain good overall hygiene. So, you have to love yourself first. Nobody else is going to take care of your health for you; nor should they! It's your body, so you must love and care for it. When it comes to self-love, keep this in mind: *Never wait to love yourself; and it's never too late to love yourself.* This means that each day, you should perform the little acts of self-love needed to keep you healthy. It also means that self-love knows no age limits; you're never 'too old' to change! Once you have self-love, you'll find it much easier to love others as well as to love the earth.

Love conquers all. Yes, it's true. So, live your life from a loving space. When you choose to live this way, your health will improve and you'll feel good now—at least most of the time! The opposite is true as well. When you choose to be healthy, you'll find that love prevails more often in your life.

"Love mends the heart, strengthens the mind and body and nourishes the soul. It's the little acts of love performed each day towards yourself and others that will keep you feeling well and help fulfill your life."
-Dr. Samuel A. Mielcarski

Loving Support

In order to feel love, you must both give and receive it. Having a loving support system around you will help you succeed in this matter. This loving support may come from your family, friends, co-workers, spiritual institutions, and the social groups with whom you associate. With modern-day technology, you can even connect with others (in real time) at the push of a button when needed. Having loving people around will keep you motivated to live a purposeful life. Remember, you're a product of your environment. So, if you want more love in your life, you must create this environment around you. How do you create it? You choose to associate with people that will provide this environment. All too often, people play the victim role. They whine and complain about how life sucks and they don't feel loved. Well, guess what? You have the power to choose love in your life. That's right! You can choose your friends, choose your job, choose your social groups, and although you can't choose your family, you can choose how you want to interact with them. Don't be a victim case; choose love instead. (Besides, CSI is busy enough. They don't need any more victim cases!)

Make sure to give as much (or even more) loving support as you receive. Others need some loving too. If you don't give love, then others can't receive it. If you don't receive love, then others can't give it. It's a two-way street. Don't be afraid to love or be loved. Surround yourself with loving people, and help to create a loving atmosphere wherever you go. Through giving and receiving of love you will feel supported in your life, which can help you feel good now!

When it comes to love, let's not forget about the planet as well. After all, it's the place where you live. Mother Earth desires to be loved. If you choose to participate in a loving and synergistic relationship with the planet, then she will reciprocate and provide for you (sometimes tenfold!); so take good care of her. Love the planet enough to cultivate it, not destroy it. Think about production, not pollution. Strive to be a symbiont, not a parasite, on this planet. Show the world your love every day.

Loving Communication

Communication is definitely a skill, as well as an art. Sometimes, it's wise to do more listening than talking. All too often, people aren't communicating at all; rather they're just waiting to talk. All people deserve respect, especially the ones with which you have close loving relationships. It's kind of ironic that sometimes, we don't always communicate in the most loving ways with the ones we feel closest to. Why is that? Well, despite the many expert opinions on this one, I feel that it's simply a matter of being fully present and connecting with our hearts first before we speak. One of the simplest ways to become present is to just breathe slow and deeply for a moment. (Sound familiar? It should—it's Link #2- Air.)

You can use the following strategy to help make this a new speaking habit: Breathe before you speak! This means that before you open your mouth to say something, first, breathe fully and deeply. You can connect with your heart by just placing a hand on your chest over your heart region. (You should do this in a very relaxed way, so as not to look like you're having a heart attack!) Breathe into your hand through your heart-center; and then, speak. This works especially well if somebody is saying something to you in a way that you don't like. Instead of the typical knee-jerk reaction where you might lose your temper and snap back at them, you can reciprocate with love and kindness instead.

Hugging vs. Drugging

When one isn't feeling well, it may be easy to reach for a certain kind of drug to get that 'quick fix' that is desired. However, I propose a new kind of approach. This prescription reads like this: *'Three-hugs-a-day can help keep ill health away.'* Sometimes, there's nothing that helps one feel more loved, than a nice big hug. Every day, shoot for giving and/or receiving at least three hugs. Why three hugs? One for the mind, another for the body, and one more for the spirit. Hugs are very powerful, as touch is another important nutrient needed to feel good now!

Many people are touch-deprived (and suffer from a 'touch deficiency'), which can lead to feelings of loneliness, depression and being disconnected. Hugs can reverse this, as they're often an instant mood lifter, energy enhancer, and grounding tool that can make one feel more vital, nourished and complete. Hugs unite and can make one feel safe and secure. After all, who doesn't like a nice hug? If or when you find that you don't want to hug, then this is a sure sign that your heart is closed down. When your heart is closed, your health will suffer. People will often try to fill the void of love with something else, such as food, drugs, television, other vices, and even conflict, instead of a hug. Many so called 'addictions' could probably be resolved with more hugging and less drugging.

Okay, so now that you know a hug can give you the pick-me-up-effect that you may need to feel better, here are some guidelines to follow when playing the hugging game.

- **Guideline #1: Permission** - Always get permission and respect another's private and personal space, especially if you don't know them too well. Permission could be verbal (you ask them) or non-verbal (an open arms posture with a smile that's well received). Sometimes with people you already know and care about, this guideline has some flexibility. For example, let's just say that your mother is in a grumpy mood for some reason, and you know that a hug would cheer her up. Even though her energy says 'stay away', you go in for the kill anyway (kill her grumpy mood that is) by giving her a big loving hug. (Note: If your mom doesn't like this, don't tell her I told you to do it, okay?)

- **Guideline #2: Time** - When a hug is meant to be over, then let go. Don't hold a person in a hug that doesn't want to be there. This can ruin the whole point of hugging. Again, you should always respect another's personal space and comfort level.

- **Guideline #3: Force** - When hugging, embrace deeply, but gently. The object is to caress somebody, not crush them. Bear hugs are usually not too comfortable. If somebody hugs you too hard, you can take a breath (hopefully), which will create some space between you, and then just let the other person know. Say something like: "I love you too, but not too hard please".

- **Guideline #4: Height** - Keep the hug at a level where your hearts can unite. If you're about the same height, then this can occur much easier. If you're the taller one, then squat down to meet the other person heart-to-heart. If you make them stand on their toes instead to reach you, they may be uncomfortable, off balance, or catch your shoulder in their throat (not fun).

- **Guideline #5: Contact** - You should make sufficient contact with the other person to make the hug feel comfortable and complete. Your upper and lower body should touch, not just your upper chests. In other words, focus on hugging the other person, not burping them. It's possible to have your upper and lower body's touching without your pelvic regions touching, which should only happen if both people are comfortable doing so. Again, respect the other person's personal space.

- **Guideline #6- Intention** - When hugging somebody, your energy and thoughts should be on love, not lust. Know who you're hugging and keep your intentions clear. You should be able to hug somebody else without becoming aroused. However, in certain situations (love-making), this may be desired by both people.

- **Guideline #7 Direction** - The direction in which you hug can make a big difference in the benefit you receive from it. Do you know which way you hug? Do you hug to your left or to your right? Does it really matter? I believe it does. Hugging to the right seems more powerful. When you hug somebody to your right (which means your chin ends up over their left shoulder), then your hearts seem to make a stronger connection. When heart energy lines up, it's a powerful experience! So, when hugging, just remember this: *'To the right, hearts unite!'* How will you really know if the direction of your hugs matter? Again, you'll have to run an experiment: compare hugging to the right versus hugging to the left, and note any differences that you feel.

*Bonus: See a video demonstrating the 'right' hugging method. Visit: FeelGoodNowTheBook.com. Enter bonus code: FGN8

The following 'Link Builder' will help you address your 'Love Link' when it needs attention. Reading or saying this phrase often can serve as a nice reminder about the importance of love to feel good now!

*Link Builder: If you want to feel good and above, then you must give and receive love!

Conclusion

Where To Go From Here To 'Feel Good Now'…
The Rest Of Your Life!

Well, if you've made it this far, then I congratulate you! I hope that you've received some very useful information to help you improve your health. At this point, I would like to review some key things with you again to help augment the learning process and guide you on your *feel good now* journey. Below are ten key reminders to help you become more successful with your goal of feeling better.

Ten Key Reminders

Reminder 1: *You have permission to change your health.* It was given to you at the beginning of this book, and you're being given it again right now! However, you don't need my permission because you get to decide your own health destiny. You just have to choose what level of health you want.

Reminder 2: *Your results will come down to two things*. First: Your willingness to learn. Hopefully, you now know what you need to do to transform your health. Second: Your willingness to change. Now, you just need to apply what you know on a consistent basis. Remember, there is a big difference between knowing (knowledge) and doing (wisdom). If you're supposed to become wiser as you get older, then why couldn't your health improve?

Reminder 3: *All habits are hard to break, not just the bad ones.* So, all you have to do is establish good habits by making small improvements each day and each week and you're bound to succeed! Your goals are not the end result you desire, but rather what's in front of you. Hopefully, you now have the guidance you need to take action to achieve your health goals (or implement what new standards you need to live by).

Reminder 4: *Mother Nature is NOT prejudiced!* This means that all who choose to live in a way that is aligned with Nature's simple guidelines will have good health. Good health is a product of healthy living. Good health can't be bought; it must be earned by providing your body, mind, and spirit with some basic needs through what I like to call: 'The Chain-of-Health System™'. Although 'Mother Nature isn't prejudiced', she is consistent with her consequences. This means that if you keep violating the rules of good health, you won't have good health. Nature has a way of making some lessons very painful. Hopefully, you're not a very slow learner!

Reminder 5: *If you want the fastest way back to better health—'the quick fix'—then you have to work on your weakest ('key') link first!* (Remember: "A chain is only as strong as its weakest link.") Now that you've read through the book, hopefully this makes much more sense. It's also important to remember that focusing more on a stronger link doesn't make up for a lack of a weaker one. For example, you can't breathe your way out of not enough sleep, or eat your way out of not enough sun, or exercise your way out of poor hygiene. Also, keep the balance between all links in the chain. No one link in your Chain-of-Health System™ is more important than the others, but certain links may require more attention at certain times.

Reminder 6: *Small steady improvements will lead to large changes in your health over time.* Consider this: Just as little as a two percent improvement per week can lead to a hundred percent improvement by the end of one year. Let's do some simple math again to help you stay motivated: 2% improvement x 52 weeks in a year = 104% improvement. (Again, you get two weeks off for good behavior!)

Reminder 7: *Chasing the 'Holy Grail of Health' can be fun, but it will lead to less than optimal results.* It's not one thing some of the time, it's many things most of the time that really works! Following a 'system of health', as opposed to relying on only one aspect of it, will give you better results in the long-run. You don't have to be perfect, but you do need to be better than you currently are now if you want better health.

Reminder 8: *The functioning of the human body is very complex; its maintenance and care should be very simple.* Follow the 'art of health' (which is simple) versus the 'science of health' (which can be complicated). The 'art of health' can be summed up with this basic mantra: 'Health comes from healthful living.' Remember: Health is earned! Just do the little things correctly each day. Keep health matters simple and you will succeed. Stick to the basics (follow the Chain-of-Health System™). There is a significant difference between 'common sense' and 'common practice'. Allow the common-sense knowledge you've gained from this book to become common practice in your life. Again, if you don't do it, then you really don't know it.

Reminder 9: *Find out what motivates you—pain or rewards (or both).* If you have a good reason to be healthy, then you will make it a worthwhile pursuit. You will find the time, spend the money, and make the sacrifices needed to be healthy. Health will become a top priority in your life.

Reminder 10: *Knowing where to start will help you end up where you want to be.* If you're not assessing, then you're just guessing. So, don't guess; assess instead! Use the Chain-of-Health System™ to help you take inventory on your health so you know where to begin to get the fastest results. After all, that is why you probably read this book in the first place—you wanted the 'quick fix'!

Chain-of-Health 'Link Builders'

Were you also hoping that I would include a page that had all of your 'Link Builders' on it to make it easier for you to find them again in the future? Well, I have you covered my 'health-seeking' friend. You can find them all below.

*Food Link: To feel good now and thrive, eat the 'fast foods' that are alive!

*Air Link: Breathe low, slow, and through the nose with lips closed!

*Water Link: Feeling down and out may be due to drought— consume more water!

*Light Link: Natural light by day is the feel good way. Artificial light by night can cause strife!

*Rest Link: If you want to feel your best, then take some R.E.S.T.!

*Activity Link: When your body starts to talk, it's time to move or take a walk!

*Hygiene Link: If you want your health to beam, then you must keep your body and living space clean!

*Love Link: If you want to feel good and above, then you must give and receive love!

As mentioned at the beginning, as well as throughout each chapter, this book offers a great way to help you *feel good now!* It does provide a 'quick fix' when you're not feeling well. When applied correctly, it may also help keep you well overall. However, will it always work? Realistically, it probably won't. Why? Health challenges can be a bit more complex than what this 'quick-fix' solution can always provide. The total scope of the essential eight links in the Chain-of-Health System™ as covered in this book aren't meant to be a cure-all, but rather a great place to begin. Why? *The solutions that are the simplest and least invasive are often the best place to start!* Of course, this is assuming that you don't have an immediate medical emergency situation that may require a more invasive approach to help save your life.

> *"Motivation is what gets you started. Habit is what keeps you going."*
> - Jim Ryan

If you're willing to consistently apply what you've learned here in this book, I do believe that you'll gain some very positive health benefits. I've seen this approach change thousands of lives and I know it can help transform your life as well. Since this book may not meet all of your needs, I would like to invite you to also explore some of my other products and services. When you want to get better at something in your life, it's often wise to have a good 'coach' to help you. If you liked this book, then I know that you'll love the other tools and products that I've made available to help meet your health and healing needs. Of course, you're probably thinking, "Okay, how much?" It really just depends on what your needs are and how much you want to invest in your health.

I have opportunities that range from free to thousands of dollars. For example, you can sign up for my blog, newsletter and YouTube Channel. You could invest in my other books, audio programs or an online course. You may desire private or group coaching services. You may want to have me come out and speak to your group or organization. Or, you may want to attend one of my week-long intensive health retreats in a tropical paradise. So, where do you go from here? There are many options. The choice is really yours. It just depends on your needs.

At a minimum, let's please stay connected via my website. It's very affordable—it's FREE! I would love to continue to help 'coach' you so that you can not only feel good now, but also feel good for the rest of your life! You can find me here: DrSamPT.com

In loving service,

Dr. Samuel A. Mielcarski, DPT (aka: 'Dr. SAM')

About The Author

You were given the gift of life. Dr. Samuel A. Mielcarski (aka 'Dr. SAM') reveals how to give yourself the gift of living well. As a speaker, author and consultant specializing in rehabilitation and health transformation, Dr. SAM has empowered thousands of people of all ages to overcome various health challenges and heal, not only their bodies, but their whole way of being. Dr. SAM's 17 years of clinical experience as a licensed physical therapist and rehabilitation expert has allowed him to gain valuable insight for guiding and coaching others towards having a better quality of life. Dr. SAM's unique system of health and healing (Chain-of-Health System™) will revolutionize the way people practice therapy as well as improve their health. This system is safe, affordable, and easy-to-follow–and it provides people with a true 'quick fix'!

Dr. SAM is a genuine role model for healthful living. He is the author of the books: 'Feel Good Now!' and 'Dr. SAM's Revolutionary Rehab Manual'; and the creator of the 'Bad Health Be Gone' health transformation program, as well as Dr. SAM's 'RAW-habilitation Health Retreats'. People often leave Dr. SAM's lectures, retreats and therapy sessions with a whole new way of thinking and appreciation about how to take charge of their health. Whether providing guidance to one individual or to many, Dr. SAM's passion for healthy living is said to be contagious. Dr. SAM is also said to have that 'magic healing touch' and has been described as: *'A clinician on a mission to help resolve the issues in your tissues'.* Dr. SAM's dedication to helping others combined with his sense of humor and practical health advice have made him a highly sought-after health and healing facilitator. Dr. SAM's guidance may not only change your life, it may even save it!

Learn more here: DrSamPT.com

26860396R00046

Made in the USA
Charleston, SC
19 February 2014